The Dark Side of Surviving Gastric Bypass Surgery

(What Doctors Don't Disclose)

Dr. Joseph A. Resnick, Ph.D.

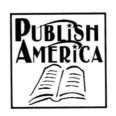

PublishAmerica
Baltimore

First printing

At the specific preference of the author, PublishAmerica allowed this work to remain exactly as the author intended, verbatim, without editorial input.

ISBN: 1-4241-6525-3
PUBLISHED BY PUBLISHAMERICA, LLLP
www.publishamerica.com
Baltimore

Printed in the United States of America

The Dark Side of Surviving Gastric Bypass Surgery

(What Doctors Don't Disclose)

Dr. Joseph A. Resnick, Ph.D.

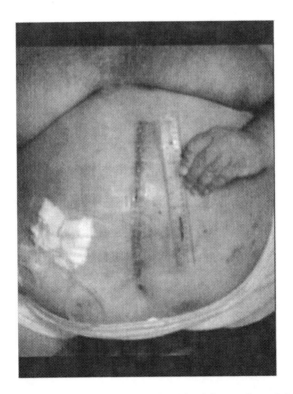

This is a photograph of the surgical incision taken thirty-six hours after radical surgery for gastric bypass procedure

Dedication and Thanks

It is with heartfelt thanks that I dedicate this book to my wife, Kathy, to my daughters, Adrienne Lynn Resnick and Nicole Yvonne Resnick, and to my grand son, Holden Austin Lane. Without their tireless love support compassion and understanding I am certain that I would not be alive today to write this book. I'd like to thank all of the persons and entities named herein for permission to use their names and thank them for the encouragement support and for that which I treasure most: Friendship. I'd like to acknowledge the medical teams that helped me to survive this ordeal, too. Without their expertise I wouldn't be here today. Thank You All!
—*Dr. Joe Resnick*

Photography Credits and Thanks

Special Thanks to Adrienne L. Resnick, Kathy Y. Resnick, Nicole Y. Resnick for photographs taken after surgery. Thanks to the National Aeronautics and Space Administration for permission to re-print the Cover of NASA Tech Briefs Magazine, September, 1994, in this book. Thanks to Mike Ramos for taking the photo of me Kathy Resnick and Jimmy Buffett in Las Vegas, NV in October, 1998 which is included in this book.

CONTENTS

Introduction

When I first considered undergoing the gastric bypass procedure I had many reservations. At that time, 1998 to 1999, the surgical technique was relatively new and data sets regarding aspects, such as survival rates, rates of patients who develop complications, etc., simply did not exist. When I, ultimately, made the decision to undergo the surgery the thought occurred to me that I might be able to help other obese people gain insight as to what they might anticipate in terms of potential experiences, by documenting my own experience from both the physical and psychological perspectives. So, I decided to memorialize my experience by making a video documentary showing what my body looked like prior to undergoing the surgery and then documenting what my body looked like as I underwent various surgical procedures lost the weight and recovered from the ordeal. It was quite an ordeal I must admit.

The DVD-documentary showing the metamorphosis is entitled, **You Can Live Again.** I would be happy to send a copy to you at no charge and for just the small fee to cover the cost of shipping and handling. To obtain a copy of the video-documentary please contact me via my web page at URL http:// www. Geocities. Com/ jreznik888.html. Alternatively, you may visit my web page at Publish America's web site (www.PublishAmerica.com) for contact information and to request a copy of the documentary. My hope is that you will benefit from witnessing the metamorphosis I underwent, both the good and the not so good.

Obesity is not something that just happens to you one day. For example you just don't go to bed one night with a normal weight and wake up the next morning and, Oh no…Boing!: You wake up and you weigh six hundred pounds! Obesity doesn't happen that way. It's a gradual and very personal thing occurring over a protracted period of time. In my opinion there are many factors contributing to the onset of obesity each of these unique to the individual. These factors may occur early in life and are enabled by psychological or life events, e.g., births, deaths, marriages, job changes, monetary issues, etc. And each of these events can impact the onset of obesity. There are likewise educational and cultural considerations which may impact clinical onset of obesity as well. For example most people just don't understand anything about nutrition. This is especially true in the case of children and adolescents. Not much time is spent educating the general public with regard to the importance of proper nutrition. At least this kind of education was not taking place when I was a kid. I surely did not understand anything about nutrition and neither did my parents nor family siblings. Of course there was the socioeconomic aspect of my childhood too. My dad died when I was eight years of age leaving mom with six kids to feed. So we ate just about anything that was not still wiggling especially less expensive foods such as potatoes which we were able to grow in our own garden. Other inexpensive fat-building foods included pasta and breads…which Mom made from scratch every couple of days. From a young age highly-glutenated foods cheap and inexpensive sources of sustenance played a role in my physical development. My belief is that through eating these kinds of foods at such an early age and over a prolonged period of time, ten to twelve years, my body was pre-conditioned to invite onset of obesity. I can recall reading some clinical data to that effect. You'll have to search that out.

In my case I can remember being the proverbial fat kid. I can recall being jided by my peers and siblings. But I never knew that I was not normal in terms of comparison of body sizes. At such an early age one has no standard for comparison other than through socialization and exposure to peer groups other people. Socialization occurs contemporaneously after the fact and after a person is already obese and the subject of ridicule and public humiliation.

After all I did not learn to read until I was about seven or eight years of age. And certainly when I was growing up during the 1960's and 1970's you were either fat skinny or someplace in between. From the time I was a child through adolescence and adulthood I battled with weight fluctuations. In grade school at around age twelve I weighed about one hundred and fifty pounds and was the heaviest kid in my school. This was one and a half times more than the other boys in my class. I used to dread the day when the doctor examined us and I had to stand in a line with all the other boys and girls and they could hear the nurse blurting out comments to the doctor like here's a fat one. In school among peers each kid strove for some kind of significance that set them apart from other kids. My distinction in addition to being the very best in my class at Science was being the heaviest kid. All the other kids knew how proficient I was at Science and I made no bones about using my weight if necessary to defend myself and my friends from older playground bullies. And I did this on several occasions defending smaller weaker classmates from upper classmen. So there was a good side to being so big. Smaller and even older kids knew I wouldn't take any bull shit from anyone. And when someone did call me fat-names I simply grabbed them pulled them to the ground and proceeded to beat the living tar out of them! They never called me fat-names again!

By the time I entered high school I weighed over two hundred pounds but I had gained height. I was nearly six feet tall by the time I finished the ninth grade. When I entered the tenth grade I was six feet tall and I was considered to be a big boy. I didn't consider myself to be fat, as such, just big. I felt okay with my size and was very popular with female classmates. And if anyone ever did make any negative comments to me about being fat or big I'd just beat them to a bloody pulp and that was the end of that. I developed quite a reputation in high school as someone you don't want to mess with. And this reputation stuck with me for the remainder of my high school years. As to the ladies I had many female friends and crushes and my reputation was that of the proverbial gentle giant. And that was true. I treated everyone with kindness. I never used my size to bully anyone and was always a gentleman to classmates to my teachers. I was taught how to love by my mom. I learned about manners and politeness at a very early age.

The first time I really noticed that I had a problem with my weight was after I graduated from high school and applied for a job with a major corporation. I passed the employment test with a score of one hundred percent. But I failed the physical examination because I was twelve pounds overweight. The maximum weight for my age-group at that time was two hundred and ten pounds for a person six feet tall. And I weighed two hundred and twenty two pounds on the day I took my employment physical. I was crushed to learn that I was not going to be hired because I was overweight. This was the first time in my life at age twenty years that I realized that weight control was a real societal issue and that I had to do something about it. I feared that I might not be able to get a job finish college and I didn't even want to think about other things like girl friends, etc. But all of these things eventually became issues in my life as I matured.

In 1974 I met and eventually married my wife, Kathy. At the time I weighed only about one hundred sixty five pounds. At that time in my life I was very active. I was in college at the University of Pittsburgh, and worked full-time as an Electrical Engineer at Westinghouse Electric Corporation in East Pittsburgh, PA. And I operated my own private real estate business through purchase of abandoned properties from the City of Pittsburgh. I spent my spare time rehabilitating these old building in order that I could rent apartments in them. I did that with a great deal of commercial success and by the time of my twenty third birth day had amassed a net worth in real estate values of just over a million dollars. I also bought some vacant land in Florida for investment purposes which I still own.

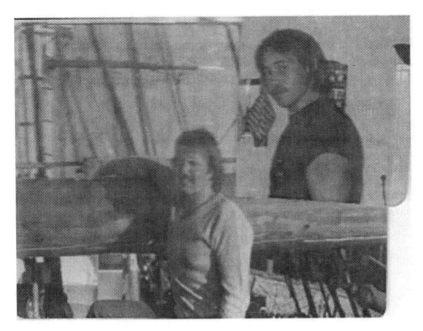

This is a photograph of me taken in 1977-78 in Florida

I never sat still never drank used dope nor anything like that. I worked full time attended college classes studied electrical and mechanical engineering in an apprentice program at Westinghouse and would spend my spare time working at one of my buildings. I taught myself how to lay flooring and carpeting learned how to wire electrical service panels and taught myself about plumbing roofing and masonry. This kind of very active lifestyle helped me keep the weight problem in check during those years. I was able to keep weight off until I suffered a broken back. As a result of that injury I stopped lifting weights playing ball and had to quit hunting and fishing. In 1979 I started to put on weight and by 1983 I had ballooned-up to over two hundred and fifty pounds. I kept that weight on for the next eight years vacillating between two hundred twenty to two hundred fifty pounds but never seeming to be able to get below two hundred and twenty pounds. I felt and looked good though and had no health problems of any kind. I never got colds or headaches and had no health issues of any kind. I felt great strong and robust just being a big or large man. I had the physique of Apollo a chest the size of Man-Mountain Dean's and forearms that looked like Popeye's! I used to be able to crack walnuts in both hands at the same time. And from a standing position I could contort my body by bending-over backwards and pick up a dime from the floor with my lips! Damn I was in good shape! I could work for twenty hours straight without a break. Eat anything that didn't wiggle. And love making episodes could carry on for hours extending into days in some cases. Damn: those were the good old days!

Obesity finally got the best of me when I was in my forties. Through my twenties and thirties I worked two jobs went to school full time in pursuit of my five college degrees; raised a family; had four cars, two boats, two vacation homes, a lovely wife, went to Disney World every year…and even managed to sneak away to Las Vegas, five to ten times a year. But the obesity finally caught up to me when I hit my forty second birthday. By the age of forty I had amassed a small fortune through sales of licenses to my patented inventions enjoyed a fabulous lifestyle had a great family life. But in retrospect I believe that being obese made me the saddest man I knew. I was unhappy with my own body image tired of being so fat and unable to do things with my wife and children. And although I appeared to be happy I was anything but. And I felt so bad for my wife because she would hear people make comments about my obesity. Things like, "Look at that beautiful woman with that fat slob. He must be rich or she's a Hooker. Otherwise she wouldn't be with him". Those kinds of comments were demeaning to both of us. But people will always be people. In a later in chapter entitled, **At the Mall,** I'll tell the story of the two men who changed my life and how I almost changed theirs too and how this encounter impacted my ultimate decision to undergo the gastric bypass procedure.

If you're reading this book you are probably suffering from Obesity just like I did. I understand that kind of suffering very well and very deeply. There are some things that happened to me that the Doctors didn't warn me about. These were physical and psychological conditions that took me completely by surprise as a consequence of undergoing the gastric bypass procedure. I don't blame the doctors for these oversights. At that time some seven years ago gastric bypass surgery was an emerging field in terms of the field of Bariatric Medicine. And the field is yet too embryonic for the doctors to have all the answers. Doctors don't have all the answers. Some day they may. My hope is that through these pages and by sharing my personal experiences you'll be spared some of the suffering I and my family have experienced. And you'll be more aware of possible risks and outcomes if you decide to undergo this kind of surgery. My belief is that you can finally overcome the stigmas associated with your obesity and that you can live again. If you decide to undergo this kind of surgical procedure don't kid yourself: It's not going to be easy. And forget words like moderate to severe discomfort. Those are sugar-coated politically-correct terms the medical profession uses for what is akin to having a hot poker shoved up you ass twisted and then yanked-out! What you're going to experience is extreme to severe pain unlike anything you've ever known in the past! I'm not talking about the kind of pain you feel with a headache. I'm talking about real pain; vomiting; seizures and blackouts from drug overdoses. That's the kind of pain I'm talking about! And at times you'll question your decisions. You'll question God and the doctors and everyone around you! You'll probably question everything you've ever held sacred. And ask yourself: What was I thinking when I made this decision to undergo this ordeal?

In retrospect it's been one hell of an ordeal. But I lived through it and I've kept the weight off for over six years. My life is much better is some ways and much worse in others. But I'm still alive and I still Rock! Many obese people were not so fortunate. Hey: Maybe you can be one of the beautiful people?

—Joseph A. Resnick, B.A., M.A., Ph.D.

Chapter 1.
Admission

I decided to name the first chapter, Admission, for the reason that I was absolutely in denial of the fact that I battled obesity for more than 20 years. I think obesity is a societal issue and agree that obesity has reached epidemic proportion in America. Consequently, before I could make the commitment to change the way I looked I had to first admit that I had a problem and recognize that I was suffering from morbid obesity. Even when I hit my fortieth birth day and weighed over three hundred pounds I still in my own mind refused to admit that I was morbidly obese. I used to joke about being so fat with my wife and kids negating my voluminous size to a perception problem. I had a vision of my own self-image which each of us has. For more information see: Cornelison, FS Jr., Dis Nerv Syst. 1963 Apr;2:133-5. No abstract available. PMID: 14023056 [PubMed - OLDMEDLINE for Pre1966]. And I liked me the way I looked the way people moved out of the way when I approached or entered an area. I liked who I was career-wise too in my community and in society. And although I knew some people made fun of me joked and made cracks about my size I tended not to let those things get to me because I was so successful in terms of my work my discoveries my inventions and my businesses. I was highly respected and sought-after by NASA, government agencies and the Department of Defense. I reasoned in my own mind that the people calling me names and making smart-ass cracks could simply kiss my ass. In my mind I believed that they were just jealous of my success and good looks. I could see jealousy on their faces as I drove away laughing all the way to the bank with twenty thousand dollars in cash carried in my socks and in a new Hummer with Alien characters painted on the side and a special license plate that read Seventy Five Grand! I figured this was not too shabby for a fat slob! And let's not forget that I had on my arm the most beautiful gal in these parts my wife, Kathy, who still rivals any Playboy Bunny I've ever seen met or had do lap dances for my friend's. All things considered I thought I was on top of the world! But I was in denial as to my obesity and was unaware of the severity of the dire risks to my health and my longevity. This attitude was another masking technique I used to hide from the fact that I was morbidly obese. Other people use other excuses and utilize some other form or masking technique. The above examples were just a few of mine. You have and masking techniques too. Think about what these may be?

People in American society have a propensity to believe that fat or obese people are inherently poor uneducated and disgusting fat slobs possessing little or no social value. The popular media adds to this societal perception through publicity of young thin females shapely models and then reinforces the underlying notion subliminally that fat people are somehow un-cool. Thus in Western Society there is a stigma associated with being obese and not conforming to what is considered to be normal body size. These biases are supported by present-day clinical publications such as that found in the Clinician's Handbook of Preventive Services, 2nd Edition: Adults and Older Adults— Screening, Chapter 29, published by the US Department of Health and Human Services (see: http://www.vnh.org/PreventionPractice/ch29.html). In other cultures such as Asia for example and in American Samoa being heavy is equated with strength superiority wealth and attractiveness. Large males are sought-after by females in those cultures. I wanted to mention these facts for your information as they were considerations for me which I encountered while making my decision to undergo the gastric bypass procedure.

I was aware of these factors the stigmas and my own encroaching physical problems and possible physical limitations. And I knew that my own realizations as to the social value of obese persons and what most people thought or believed was simply not true. I felt that despite my obesity I had social worth and contributed to the forward progress of Mankind through my work, my inventions and my discoveries. After all I was a five hundred pound Millionaire with the Midas touch on top of my game personally and professionally. And the fact that I was obese had absolutely nothing to do with my personal achievements leading to personal attainment of socioeconomic status and wealth. I reasoned that society and these ignorant people were all simply wrong about fat and obese people. It's very difficult for one to try to overcome societal views and stigmas let alone engender to challenge them. Disabled people, amputees and people who must use wheel chairs, for example, know this experience all too well. Obese people live with constant humiliation and stereotyping, too. The stereotyping is a societal thing engrained in the American culture and Western Society. If you're overweight you're automatically considered to be worthless to society assumed to be uneducated probably with no money living on Welfare and projected to ultimately end up being a burden to society and a ward of the state. On the other hand if you're tall thin and even moderately good looking you get the best jobs live in the best neighborhoods drive the nicest cars etc. These notions are supported by the popular press and some of the professions as well by virtue of publication of qualified and quantified data.

Even with all those givens and realizing the cognitive dissonance in the comparisons I still was in denial that I was obese. I had excuses for my size and I even made up a few things. And sometimes when confronted by family members, who would ask me about my health, how I felt, and certainly out of love for me would ask if they could help me lose weight, I was evasive. In some instances I even became maddened and severed life-long relationships with these family members. From the perspective related to health issues and obesity, my family members were correct and the things they did and said were done and mentioned out of love for me not viciousness. And I made mistakes by severing relationships as I thought they were against me and not for me. I felt that they should love me, regardless of my body size. After all they sure did say they loved me when I handed them a check for twenty or twenty five thousand dollars.

My family members could see the pain I felt. Like the time one of the airlines insisted that I purchase two seats because I was so large and so fat. I was humiliated! If I would have had access to another five or ten million dollars I'd have tendered an offer to purchase that airline just so that I could shut it down and fire everybody that worked for it. Bitter? You bet your boots! But I'm smart enough to know that I couldn't fight dragons! So I just released that bitterness.

In 1995 I took my wife, lab assistant and a close friend with me for a mini-vacation to Las Vegas, Nevada. When we were checking in the ticket agent made a comment about my weight and asked me how much I weighed. The fellow blurted out his question within ear-shot of all standing in the long ticket lines. I was mortified. When I answered his query he stated that I would have to purchase two seats because I was so large. When that happened to me I became really angry and I was humiliated. Not knowing how to react I simply bought-out every available seat in the First Class section. I purchased all available twenty seats. I invited every fat person on that flight to join me and those in my party. There were eight fatties in the waiting area. When we finally boarded and the plane was loaded I had the stewardesses draw the curtains in front and back of the First Class compartment and I made and posted signs that read: FAT PEOPLE AND GUESTS ONLY— NO SKINNY PEOPLE WELCOME. On the ground I bought the first round of drinks for everyone in the cabin to get everyone primed for the seven hour flight to LAV. After takeoff and leveling off at twenty six thousand feet we started to order food and drinks from the two stewardesses assigned to the First Class cabin. Including me and my two guests there were twelve people in First Class and a remaining eight empty seats which I had purchased. We started ordering more drinks and food, which were free in First Class, and we proceeded to eat all of the food in the ship's pantry and we drank their bar dry before we hit McCarran Air Port! The airline lost money that day despite my having paid almost four thousand dollars for those extra seats. Our party drank more than one hundred thirty of those little bottles of booze and we each had five or six sandwiches. We consumed five trays of fruit and cheeses, drank 9 bottles of wine, and ate 36 dinners! Neither the money nor the cost mattered to me. I had plenty of money. I guess I was trying to prove a point to the airline. They won, in terms of my compliance with policy requiring obese people to purchase two seats. But I know they lost money on that flight from the cost of the food and beverage services consumed by this little group. Eventually, the Captain came into the cabin and apologized to me. I was gracious, although thoroughly shit-faced by the time he came back and I offered to buy him a drink! I have not flown on that airline since. I'll never fly that airline again in this lifetime.

With all of that said I finally admitted to myself that I was morbidly obese and that I had to do something about it. I began to explore options and various ways in which I might begin to lose the weight I needed to lose. I needed to lose almost four hundred pounds!

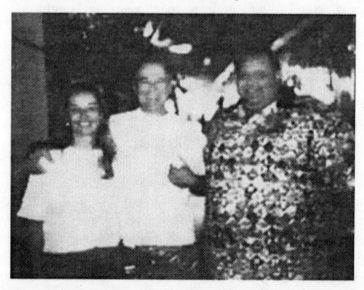

Above is a picture of what I used to look like when we made that trip to Vegas. My wife, Kathy, and friend, Jimmy Buffett, are in the photo with me (I'm the 'Fat Guy')! This photograph was taken back stage at the MGM Grand Hotel in October, 1998.

Chapter 2.
Weight Loss Programs

In 1998 I became very concerned about my size and the fact that my weight was rapidly approaching four hundred pounds. Despite my reduction of food intake and even starting an exercise regime which I practiced every day at home, at work, etc. I couldn't lose any significant amount of weight. One would think or have a tendency to believe that morbidly obese people would have to ingest large amounts of food, daily, just to maintain the weight level or to maintain such a large body mass. That was not the case with me. During a typical day my caloric intake rarely exceeded five hundred to a thousand calories. A typical day in my routine consisted of arising at six A.M. shower shave and walk out the door. I would arrive at my office and lab by seven A.M. At the lab I would make a pot of coffee and I never ate any breakfast. Over the course of the morning from seven A.M. to Noon I would drink two or three cups of coffee with cream and no sugar. I never drank any kinds of soda-pop and I never ate lunch. While my staff was at lunch I would take long walks in the community park in Brackenridge, PA. The community park was located across the street from my office-lab and which ran along the Allegheny River from Tarentum, PA to Natrona, PA a distance of about two miles. At lunch time regardless of the climate conditions I would spend an hour walking briskly in the park along the river-walk. I used to enjoy this routine and even looked forward to it. To supplement my walking exercises my wife purchased a heavy-duty rebounder for me to use at my lab. I kept this device in my office. During the course of the day when I became bored or needed a break from my work, which was sedentary, I would use the rebounder device to undertake run-in-place exercises, stair-step exercises, etc. And I would do this several times through the course of a typical day and in the afternoons before leaving my office.

At around two o'clock every afternoon I would drink a bottle of water and eat a piece of fruit. Generally I kept fruit in my office. I would share the fruit with my parrot, Nikko, which I kept caged in my Office. Generally I'd give half of the apple to Nikko just to shut him up! I made a very conscious effort to lose weight for more than a year to no avail. It seemed that the more I tried to lose weight the more weight I gained. Routinely I'd leave the office-lab at around three o'clock in the afternoon and I'd be home within seven minutes or so. I had my travel routine down to a science!

My wife always had a dinner prepared for our family. Typically dinner was served promptly at five o'clock. My wife who's a great cook always prepared health-conscious meals for our family consisting chiefly of fish foul and occasionally trimmed red meats. We had red meats only occasionally as our daughters did not like to eat red meats. We always had plenty of fresh veggies salads with vinegar dressings and low calorie drinks. I had a great support system in place in terms of my family's active efforts to help me lose weight. And I realized that if I was going to live another fifteen to twenty years that I absolutely had to lose the excess weight.

Chapter 3.
Support Groups and Support Systems

Just a brief word about support groups and support systems. Some people considering undergoing the gastric bypass procedure may lack support systems in their lives or at home or in their families. I had a very strong support system in the form of my immediate family and felt that I did not need to take advantage of the support group meetings which were offered by the hospital where I had my surgery. Adding to my decision not to utilize those support systems were the facts that I really distrusted some of the clinicians who purported to be experts regarding the prospect of surviving gastric bypass surgery. My logic was to question how these skinny little women who had those petite little bodies could ever have any inkling of how I might have felt what I was thinking or what it was like to weigh five or six hundred pounds? They could not have known how I felt or what it was like to weigh almost six hundred pounds.

Clinics and hospitals have support groups and professional counselors available to help the prospective patients with questions, concerns, etc. In my particular situation I did not feel that I needed to utilize the services of such available services and professionals. My particular situation was pretty cut and dried: Have the surgery lose the weight or die a horrible death from complications due to my obesity.

There's a good chance that if you're reading this book you're considering undergoing the gastric bypass procedure. If that's the case be aware of the availability of support groups support systems counselors, etc. Where ever you decide to have you surgery done you should be aware of the value of using these services. Since the time that I had my surgery six years ago many advances have been made and the knowledge base regarding this kind of surgery has evolved and come into being. At the time I had my surgery much of this new knowledge simply did not exist. It does now. I recommend that you consider taking advantage of the advancements in areas of the Social Services which have been made. Don't be afraid to ask questions about anything. No question is stupid especially where your life and well being is concerned. If you need help ask for it. If you want counseling demand it! If you have pain do whatever you have to get the attention you need to stop the pain! Make no mistake about it. There's going to be lots and lots of pain.

In late 1998 while on a vacation with my family in Atlantic City, New Jersey, I was bitten by a Brown Recluse Spider on the lower right leg (calf) while sleeping in a hotel room. This happened while I was asleep. When I awakened in the morning the lower portion of my calf had swollen to the size of a basketball and I could not pull my pants over my calf. I immediately called my doctor in Pittsburgh, and we headed for the hospital straight away. It took us 6 hours to drive back to Pittsburgh, from Atlantic City. We dropped our kids off at the house and my wife took me right to the hospital where I was admitted as an in-patient. I spent five days in the hospital suspended with IV's in both arms. I laid in that hospital bed waiting to see if the Propicillen could stop the infection and necrosis in the extremity and praying that the gangrene would not set in resulting in possible amputation of the limb. I was fortunate. The antibiotics took effect and I did not lose the leg. But even while a patient and hospitalized believe it or not and to my utter astonishment I gained nearly thirty pounds in that five day period. Over the time period I had not eaten a thing. I drank a few cups of ice water and drank one can of ginger ale. My primary care physician attributed the weight gain to the IV's but I knew better. I counted each bag every drop from each of the two of the IV-drips and over the duration the IV's could not have delivered more that two gallons of liquid. At most this would have been sixteen pounds of liquid. I was voiding regularly and there were no problems with my kidneys. So I did the math and determined that at most I was given intravenously and in water-weight was no more than sixteen pounds of fluid. Yet I gained almost thirty pounds in five days. I was worried and convinced in my own mind that there was some other pathology within my body responsible for this continued weight gain. Something was causing me to gain weight and keep it on despite lack of food intake. I was not eating anything of substance and certainly less than one thousand calories per day yet I continued to gain weight!

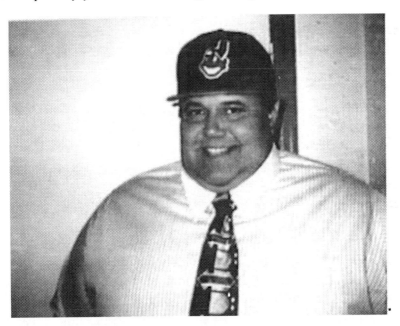

This is a picture of what I looked like in 1998 at 450 Pounds. This picture was taken in my State Room aboard the HMS Queen Mary in November, 1998 in Long Beach, CA at the "Invention Convention". The cap I am wearing contains one of my invention's, the Paparazzi-Stopper (Photographic Counter-Measure Device and Method, Patent Pending) which was featured in a Cover Story in the LA Times in November, 1998.

In early 1999 I subjected to a battery of diagnostic tests ranging from CT-scans to Smack-Thirty Two blood examinations. The hematological studies all came back negative. And unfortunately I was so fat that the CT scanners proved to be ineffective in terms of producing any studies of value to the doctors. In one case I encountered a technician who made a derogatory comment about my size expressing her concern that I was simply too fat for the machine and that I would get stuck inside of it. The technician stated her feat that I might cave-in the patient slide-platform and she refused to do a second study on me. Again, I felt the sting of humiliation and embarrassment due to my obesity. I ended up walking out of that clinic after I expressed my dissatisfaction with the technician's comments how un-professional, non-compassionate and inconsiderate that I felt she truly was. Before I left there I stated to the woman: "Yes, I'm fat. But I can lose this weight. You're always going to be ugly!" I left that place vowing never to return.

So, this was another mental defeat for me as I had hoped to discover through those tests and studies exactly what it was in my body that was preventing me from losing the weight. I didn't give up. Rather, I found a new determination and made a new commitment to myself and my family to keep going and not to give up! I didn't have a choice. Lose the weight or die.

There was another fat guy who was bigger than me who used to live in Tarentum, PA. His name was Jim. He was one of the nicest, kindest human beings I had ever encountered in my lifetime. I used to see him around town every once in a while. One time when I saw him at a local Flea Market someone made a fat comment about him. When that happened I saw the embarrassment on his face and I shared his humiliation. We joked about how some people are just ignorant and we laughed it off. I was saddened to pick up the newspaper about six months later and to read in the Obituary Column that Jim had passed away. Later I saw a mutual friend who told me that Jim had developed Diabetes as a result of the obesity and that he had to have both legs amputated and that he suffered terribly before his death. Jim developed an infection and subsequently died from those complications. I knew that he died from complications directly resulting from his obesity. As I mentioned above Jim was one of the nicest kindest and gentlest men I had ever met or known. I had known him for more than thirty years and in all those years he was always either overweight or downright obese. Consequently he was never able to gain any meaningful employment status in the nearby towns and he had no medical insurance. In the end it was obesity that killed Jim and the fact that he was unable to acquire medical care, I believe. The situation and events with Jim stuck in my mind and still does to this day. And I ponder how many obese people die every year as a result of the stigmas associated with obesity and not receiving the proper medical care needed to deal with these problems? I don't know and can't say as I am unable to find anything in the literature about this. In any event I wanted to share this with my reader's in the hope that if you're in that situation do something about it! For the love of God don't let yourself end up like Jim!

Over the course of the next few months I tried several weight loss programs to no avail. In fact, undertaking and participating in these popular programs actually resulted in my gaining more weight. This was probably due to eating pre-packaged foods that contained extraordinarily-high salt content. My opinion is that the salt in those foods added to water retention in my body and may have led to my development of edema in my extremities. I cut those programs out after about a month after my legs started swelling-up. I knew these kinds of programs simply were not for me and probably not good for other morbidly obese individuals. I started to examine other options and to search for other ways to lose the weight.

Chapter 4.
A New Hope

On a beautiful Sunday morning in the spring of 1998 I watched a television program on a local Pittsburgh TV station about a new medical procedure called Gastric Bypass Surgery. This new medical procedure was designed for morbidly obese people and persons with eating disorders and involved what was being described as a relatively safe although new surgical procedure. The story stated that this new technique was being performed at the Presbyterian University Hospital at the University of Pittsburgh by a young surgeon named Dr. Philip Schauer. I only caught a few minutes of the broadcast but I decided that I would contact the hospital the following day and get more information about the program.

The following Monday morning I continued to follow my regular routine. I would leave for work at seven o'clock in the morning and would arrive at my laboratory in Brackenridge, PA around seven twenty. At nine A.M. that morning I telephoned the main telephone switchboard at the University of Pittsburgh which I had memorized some years before while a student/teacher there and asked to be connected to Dr. Schauer's program office. Apparently, the new program was being undertaken through the Department of Minimally-Invasive Surgery at Presbyterian University Hospital's Eating Disorders Clinic. The operator put me right through to the unit secretary. When I was connected I identified myself and asked to schedule an appointment to see Dr. Schauer. My request was accommodated and an appointment was set for the following week.

My first visit to the clinic was less than enjoyable. When I arrived at the hospital I had to walk almost a mile from the parking area just to get to the main hospital entrance. Then I had trouble locating the suite of offices where the Minimally-Invasive Surgical Unit was located. And of course amid the search I was hearing the never-ending fat-comments from all manner of people: Hospital Staff, passers-bye, etc. When I finally found the offices I checked in with the unit secretary gave her my insurance cards which she returned after copying them and was invited to have a seat and told that the doctor would see me shortly. I looked around at the waiting room area and started to snicker as the chairs looked like they were salvaged from Romper Room or from a Kindergarten. They were so small and I knew I'd never be able to sit in any one of them. There were no couches nor benches nor any furniture that might accommodate a person of my size. I looked back at the secretary and queried: "Ma'am. Is this a clinic for fat people? Where do you expect me to sit? I can't sit in one of those baby chairs?". The secretary stated that the clinic was newly established and that quite frankly no one had even thought about furniture to accommodate the obese clients. I replied: "Ma'am...if this is going to be a clinic where your clients are obese people, such as myself, you'd better get some furniture so that fat guys like me can sit and wait for the doctor". I continued: "There's no place for me to sit and wait and I just walked almost a mile to get here and I'm exhausted. I'll wait another five minutes. If the doctor's not out here in five minutes I'm outta' here". The secretary thanked me. I waddled, sweating, into the room and found an empty wall against which to lean and to rest. Within the five minute time window I was called back to another waiting-exam area where I was able to sit and wait to see the doctor. Within a few minutes Dr. Schauer came into the exam room with two other people a man named Bill and a nurse named Beth. I was not in the best frame of mind for the initial meeting. I was mad as hell about the furniture incident and the fact that it took me so long to find the clinic, park, walk half a mile, get insulted along the way, and then be embarrassed because the furniture was inadequate. I explained all of this to the doctor.

In retrospect I guess I made an Ass of myself. But the doctor was very considerate of my feelings. He apologized explaining that the clinic was brand new and I was assured that the next time I visited the clinic there would be furniture there to accommodate me and other persons like me.

After we broke the ice Dr. Schauer explained the program to me. I was told that before I could be considered to be a patient-candidate for this new kind of surgery that I would have to undergo a psychological evaluation to determine whether or not I was suited for participation in the program and for the surgery. Further, that I would need to meet with a nutritionist to be evaluated. I was directed to schedule an appointment with a psychologist and with a nutritionist both of whom were members of Dr. Schauer's staff. I was told that after I was evaluated and if it were determined that I could benefit from having the surgery I would be contacted and another appointment would be scheduled at which time additional details for the proposed surgical procedure would be provided. The first time I met with Dr. Schauer I weighed in at 430 Pounds. For information on pre-screening for LRGB see: http://www.obesityresearch.org/cgi/content/abstract/13/2/234 on the World Wide Web.

Within two weeks after the first visit to meet with Dr. Schauer I scheduled and kept appointments with the psychologist who administered the Minnesota Multi-Phasic Personality Index or MMPI to me. I also met with the nutritionist. The meeting with the psychologist was cut and dried. I took the MMPI test as instructed and the results were sent to Dr. Shauer. The meeting with the nutritionist on the other hand was not very enjoyable. When I discussed my situation and eating habits with the nutritionist she challenged what I was stating in terms of my daily caloric intake and stopped just short of calling me a liar. I was very much offended by this person. She made me feel so uncomfortable and ashamed of being obese! She made accusatory statements to the effect that I must be hiding the Snickers bars under my bed and sneaking food when no one was around. Immediately I objected to this attitude on the part of this so-called professional. That encounter with this so-called expert convinced me that the nutritionist pardon the vernacular did not know shit from apple butter! I didn't find the experience with the nutritionist to be of much value and I avoided her at every chance in subsequent undertakings at the hospital and in the clinic. In fact, I never spoke with her again after that initial encounter. And this negative encounter with the nutritionist resulted in my decision not to participate in support group activities post surgery and was directly responsible for my refusal to participate in anything in which she had a hand including support groups and seminars. I mention in passing that this nutritionist has managed to gain national prominence on a national television morning program presenting as the consummate expert with regard to nutrition and health. I get a kick out of watching her pontificate during sugar-coated scripted interviews knowing that about fifty million people are watching and listening as she attempts to spoon-feed concocted data to the audience. Despite that recognition my opinion remains that this person still does not know shit from apple butter about obesity as it relates and related to my physiology and pathologies.

Obese people especially when they take such a dramatic step as to commit to have this kind of potentially life-threatening surgery need support and encouragement: They don't need criticism! I never saw any of the reports that either the psychologist or the nutritionist may have authored about me. I saw the nutritionist only one time and for less than three minutes and in that three minute time period she did more damage to me than the doctor's scalpel. After her remarks I made my decision about her so-called expertise. When I questioned her credentials she was evasive and replied with a how-dare-you-question-me attitude. I saw the psychologist only one time and for less than two minutes on the day I scheduled to meet him and take the MMPI test. When I did visit his office at the scheduled time and date he handed the MMPI test to me and told me he was late for another appointment. I was instructed to leave the completed test on his desk when I was finished. He stated that that Dr. Schauer's office would be in touch with me and again stated that he was late for a lunch-meeting and had to leave. So, there was no follow-up with neither the psychologist nor nutritionist even after I had my surgery. I'll discuss this matter in another chapter.

What the Doctors Didn't Tell Me

Finally, a word in defense of the individuals named above. At the time I entered Dr. Schauer's program it was embryonic and I was, perhaps, only the twentieth or thirtieth patient to be considered for the surgery. And according to Doctor Schauer I was the largest body weight patient ever to be considered for this kind of surgery at five hundred sixty pounds. There may have been one other man who was heavier than me but he died during surgery. Thus, I consider myself to be very, very lucky to be alive. And, admittedly, I was not the ideal patient. I questioned everything the clinicians were telling me. I questioned their educational backgrounds, challenged their expertise, demanded to know about their own experiences, etc. I guess I was a real rectum-pump at times. Okay I admit it: I was an Asshole! Dr. Schauer and I discussed this and he understood how I felt about some things how unhappy I was. He understood the societal pressures I dealt with routinely. And most importantly he commiserated with the psychological and physiological aspects of my obesity. Dr. Schauer is a very enlightened individual and expert in what he does. And there's a compassionate side to him that made me feel completely confident in him and the Program particularly in view of the fact that he was the man in charge. I took all of that into consideration when making my decision to place my life in this man's hands. And, I never questioned the competency of any member of Dr. Schauer's staff. Rather, I realized that people have bad days are very busy at times and I was not exactly the most pleasant person to deal with at that time in my life either. I was suffering. I was frightened. And I so wanted to live again!

In my second meeting with Dr. Schauer sure enough there was new furniture in the clinic and my second visit went a lot more smoothly. Dr. Schauer told me that based on the MMPI I was considered a candidate for the bypass surgery and the procedure was described to me in more detail, I was provided with some written information about the procedure describing what I could expect in terms of some of the risks and possible outcomes. Here is a link to a URL on the internet which describes the procedure Dr. Schauer performed on me. See: http://

www.laparoscopy.com/obesity/roux.html . By that time it was now June of 1999 and I decided that I would have the surgery in September.

The summer came and went and I was preparing myself psychologically and otherwise to undergo the surgery. I was cognizant of how risky the surgery would be for a man of my size. And there was the real possibility that I might not survive or that I could have some complications as a result of the surgery such as infection etc. I spent the remainder of the summer and the fall of 1999 enjoying my family my home and my friends. I got rid of my Hummer sold my laboratory donated all of my equipment. These included my favorite pieces of equipment: A Jeole 100X Phase Scanning Electron Microscope and a 12-Channel Grass Polygraph. These were donated to my favorite educational philanthropies, The Northern Westmoreland County Vo-Tech School in New Kensington, PA and to the Rhine Research Institute for Paranormal Research at Duke University in Durham, NC, respectively. In essence I was preparing for the worst and hoping for the best.

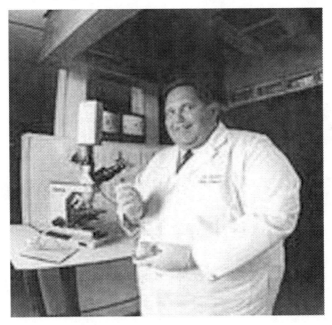

Above is a photograph of me at my Laboratory in Brackenridge, PA in 1998. My weight at that time was approximately 425 Pounds.

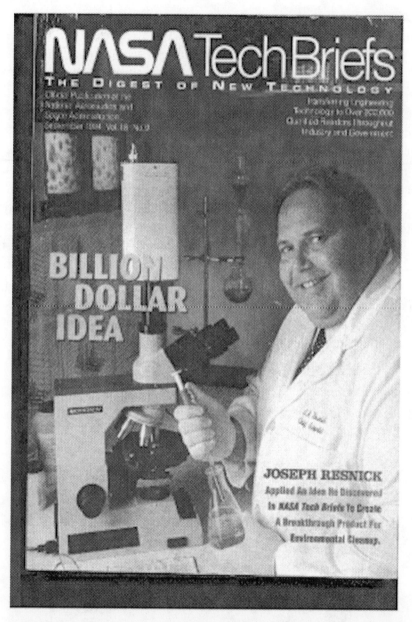

Above is a photograph of me appearing on the Cover of NASA's
Tech Briefs Magazine in September, 1994. I weighed about 360
Pounds in this photograph. (Photo used by permission from NASA HQ)

Chapter 5.
Not My Throat!

I finally got my business affairs in order and I was psyched to have the bypass surgery undertaken. I scheduled to have the surgery performed at the Presbyterian University Hospital in Pittsburgh, with Dr. Schauer leading the surgical team. The surgery was scheduled to take place in September, 1999.

Several days prior to my appearing at the pre-determined day and date for the surgery I had some bad vibes about the whole thing. My wife and I were discussing things about possible outcomes and how our lives might change based on positive or negative results. I just had a bad feeling about the whole situation. In the time that passed over the summer and fall I had attempted to contact people at the Clinic in order to get more information about the surgical procedure to no avail. I made phone calls to the psychologist and nutritionist in order to discuss some issues with them with no success. I spent hours and hours on the World Wide Web reading everything I could find out about this new surgical procedure. But in all honesty the procedure was so radically new and not much information was available even on the World Wide Web. I knew that my options were limited and that if I did not have this surgery and get rid of this weight I probably wouldn't see my fiftieth birthday.

Despite my own reservations I presented on the day and date at Presbyterian University Hospital in order to undergo the surgery. From the moment I arrived at the hospital at six A.M. I had the feeling that something was all wrong. Call it Karma or intuition or Gamut: I had the feeling that something was wrong. I just did not feel right about the situation. When I checked in at the hospital's registration desk the intake person had no record of my having an appointment to have surgery that day. I felt like an idiot standing there as the panoply of confusion among the nursing staff and administration played out before me. I immediately interpreted this as a big red flag. I expressed these concerns to these concerns to my wife and daughters.

Finally, I was taken to the pre-surgical preparation suite located in the basement of the hospital. From the moment I entered the suite I sensed pandemonium, disorder, disorganization and almost an atmosphere of utter chaos. No one seemed to know what was happening nor did I have a sense of who might be in charge of the unit. I had worked in hospitals and emergency rooms while a student at the University of Pittsburg. And possessing a Master's Degree in Public Health Management I had a very good understanding of hospital protocols. I noticed that the immediate staff was comprised mostly young females who looked to be in their late teen years or early twenties, at best. And these nurses were complaining about working conditions the time of day and how inconvenient their work hours were and how hard they had partied the night before. All of this seemed so dysfunctional and out of the ordinary to me that I was highly agitated and alarmed. My wife and daughters were with me only for a few moments just long enough to see a young lady put a wrist band on me as help me get out of my street clothes and into a gown. My wife and daughters took my clothes and put them into a bag. I climbed onto a gurney kissed my wife and daughters and said my good byes. When I was wheeled into the pre-op waiting area a nurse came in and insisted that I take off my robe and underwear. I resisted asking for a sheet or blanket. She was adamant and I complied. I demanded that she provide me with a sheet or something with which to cover myself as I was pre-nade in front of other patients and these young nurses. I later found out these young people were not nurses, rather, only students and should not have been in the surgical suite without a doctor being present. I overheard several of these staff members making jocular comments about how fat I was, and yes, there was even some laughter. This disturbed me greatly. As I lay on the gurney pre-nade and shivering an oriental woman approached me and started cackling in broken English. Frankly I could not understand a word she was saying. I had not yet been given any sedatives which I was told that I would receive in order to prepare me for the surgery. I asked this cackling oriental woman to identify herself to me. I wanted to know who she was and what she intended to do to me. Through the broken English-speak I ascertained that her name was Dr. Yee. The woman stated to me: "I Doctor Yee. I cut your throat and put in tube". At that very moment I overheard the young nurses break out into loud laughter and this frightened me very much! I stated to Dr. Yee: "Wait a minute lady. Nobody's cutting my throat! I have not been given any sedatives. I am fully aware of what's going on here and from what I can see you people don't know what the hell's going on in here! You're not touching me and you're sure as Hell not cutting my throat while I'm awake. And no one's operating on me today." The woman replied: "No-no…I cut you throat, now…you get operation". I really became frightened and informed the lady and all staff members standing around the gurney that if they did not stand away and let me off the gurney that I would kick them all and that I wanted out of that place and that no one was touching me. I made it clear that no one was cutting my throat without anesthesia! At that point and bare-ass naked all 560 Pounds of me jumped off that gurney and with my fat butt exposed to everyone I walked down the hallway until I found a sheet lying on another gurney. I wrapped it around my body and walked to the family waiting room area. My wife and daughters were shocked to see me. I told them what I had just experienced. I got dressed and then we proceeded to leave that hospital.

On the way out of the hospital as Fate would have it we ran into Dr. Schauer on the elevator while he was on his way to the Operating Room. He asked me what the problem was. And I was so traumatized that I told him that I had decided that I was not having the surgery done that day that I would write a letter to him explaining the events and reasons for my sudden departure and that he'd have the letter in a couple of days. I was nice to him and gentlemanly. I abruptly excused myself and left that hospital never to return to have surgery at that hospital.

The next day I wrote a letter to Dr. Schauer and to the Administrator at the Presbyterian University Hospital detailing the events of the encounter with the laughing staff members. I described in great detail the humiliation I endured the un-professionalism of the nursing staff and the encounter with Dr. Yee who had planned to cut my throat.

I waited for about a week to pass. I felt that amount of time to be sufficient for Dr. Schauer to have received and read my letter. I contacted Dr. Schauer's office and scheduled another office visit. I met with Dr. Schauer about a week later at which time we discussed the events at Presbyterian University Hospital. After some discussion I was satisfied with Dr. Schauer's explanation for the events at the first hospital. We agreed to re-schedule the surgery to take place at another hospital where Dr. Schauer was on staff. That hospital was Shadyside Hospital which is also part of the University of Pittsburgh Medical Center or UPMC Health System and where Dr. Schauer was also on staff. I was adamant about not having surgery at Presbyterian University Hospital. A second surgery date was scheduled at Shadyside Hospital. Dr. Schauer apologized for the events that occurred at Presbyterian University Hospital. I accepted his apology and his assurances that this would not happen again. We shook hands and I told him I'd see him pre-op on the designated day, date and time.

Chapter 6.
At the Mall...

After the negative turn of events at the first hospital and despite promising that I'd have the surgery as agreed I still had some reservations about the whole surgery-thing. It was now October, 1999 a couple of weeks before Halloween. I had hoped to have the surgery and be up and around by Halloween as this season is one of my favorite times of the year.

Halloween is one of my favorite holidays. About a week before my scheduled surgery date my wife and I decided to visit the local shopping mall in order to purchase candy and to do a little window shopping in preparation for the Christmas season. So, we jumped in the Hummer and headed to the Mall for what we thought would be a good time and perhaps even some fun.

We arrived at the Mall parked the Hummer and headed inside. At that time my weight had ballooned-up to over 400 Pounds and I used to wear sweat pants all the time as this was the only kind of clothing that would fit my eighty four inch waist. Admittedly I was down-right obese! Despite that I was in a good mood and my wife wanted to look at some new furniture. We decided to visit the furniture store first to see if there was any new furnishing that my wife might be interested in purchasing. From the furniture store we planned to hit the candy store and load-up on the Halloween candy and head back home.

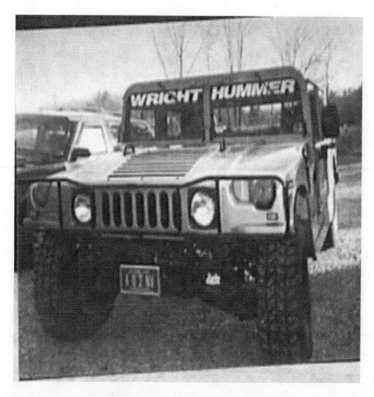

Above is a photo of the Hummer my wife and daughters bought for me as a gift on my 45th Birthday. The front license plate read in Anagram: "For You To Envy" (4 U 2 NV). At the time I owned this vehicle I weighed almost 500 Pounds and had trouble getting in and out of it.

As we entered the Mall we passed a pond that has a bridge and a fountain and some foliage displayed. There were two older men standing on the bridge apparently talking to one another. The men were in their late sixties I guessed as they both had gray hair were missing several teeth and were wearing ball caps. We had to walk past them to get to the furniture store. As we walked past them one man said to the other: "Look at that fat slob with that babe". The other man replied within earshot and loud enough for me and my wife to hear their conversation's..."She's probably a whore or a hooker. No normal woman would have anything to do with something that looks like that".

My wife heard their statements too and I stopped just for a second as I was embarrassed and humiliated for my wife having to hear something so vile and disrespectful. I hesitated at that second as I for a moment felt like pulling out my .45 caliber semi-automatic pistol and just blowing them away! I wanted to say something to them to confront them. My wife tugged at my arm and said, "Joe. Please. C'mon. Just ignore them". I complied with my wife's request and kept walking toward the furniture store. As we continued to walk the two old men continued to heckle us and make fat comments about me and derogatory things about my wife. Big mistake!

I accompanied my wife into the furniture store where she proceeded to look around for some new furniture for our game room. I told her that I had to go to the bathroom and that I would return shortly and that she should continue to look around. As I was leaving her side I said in an Arnold Schwarzenneger-Terminator-voice: "I'll be back". I think she knew what I was intending to do.

I walked out of the furniture store and made a bee-line directly for the fountain/bridge where the two old men were still standing. As I approached them from a blind side I noticed that they were heckling other passers-bye. I walked up to them and announced and said: "Gentlemen! This is your Lucky Day!" They looked at one another and the older one said to me, "What the hell do you mean?" At that point I opened my jacket and produced Rosco: A nickname I assigned to my .45 caliber semi-automatic pistol. I again stated: "This is your Lucky Day because I could kill you both where you stand right now if I want to". I continued, "I don't know what kind of Hogs you both had for Mothers but apparently they never taught you to respect a lady and to have compassion for people with disabilities. I oughtta' kill both of you old bastards right now right where you stand!" At that point one of the old men passed out and fell backwards into the fountain. The other man urinated in his pants. From behind me came my wife. My wife grabbed me by the arm and pulled me out of the Mall back to the Hummer. I was super pissed off at those two old farts! We got in the Hummer. I started it and proceeded to drive toward the exit in the parking lot. As we pulled out on to the main highway an ambulance was pulling into the parking lot main entrance at the other end of the mall. The next day in the local newspaper a story appeared telling of an incident at the local mall. The story reported that an elderly shopper lost his balance and fell into the fountain-pond at the Highlands Mall. The article said the man apparently lost consciousness while crossing the bridge in the display. The Moral of this story is: Keep your mouth shut and don't make fun of fat people. The next fat guy that you heckle might be crazier than I was at that time and that fat guy might pull the trigger!

After that event at the Mall I knew without a doubt that I had to have that surgery. In a sense the encounter with those two old farts was the proverbial straw in this camel's back. I suppose I owe them some marginal debt of gratitude. As after that encounter I was determined more than ever to proceed with the gastric bypass surgical procedure.

Chapter 7.
The Surgery

I presented at Shadyside Hospital on the scheduled day and date mentally, physically and spiritually prepared for the endeavor and for all I was about to endure. This time, at Shadyside, the staff was waiting for me and I received the real 'VIP-treatment'. The staff was so nice, so highly professional, and this did much to assuage what concerns I still maintained about having the surgery.

I was introduced to the Anesthesiologist who spent about 20 minutes with me discussing the chemicals, flow rates, etc., he planned to use during the procedure. I really appreciated this, being a 'technical-guy', with backgrounds in Chemistry and Medicine. So, I was confident that the Anesthesiologist was competent and that he was not going to over-dose me...or under-dose me, and that I was not going to awaken in the middle of a procedure with my guts spilled out all over the operating table! I have to state in retrospect that due to the excellence of this practitioner I never felt any pain. I felt no pain of any kind prior to or during the actual surgery. And for this I remain most grateful. I can't remember his name but he was definitely the best and hand-selected by Dr. Schauer.

I can recall being on the operating table as I had to help the technicians move my body onto the table. I was too fat for them to move. I can recall the Anesthesiologist stating my weight being at 564 Pounds. I couldn't believe it myself. And then I recall Dr. Schauer looking in my eyes and asking if I was okay and ready to go? I stated, "Yes…let's do it". So the fourteen-hour long procedure commenced.

It is/was my understanding that the initial procedure commenced attempting to use the minimally-invasive surgical procedure. But due to the fact that I was so large the instruments were not long enough to adequately reach my internal organs and a radical surgical procedure had to be performed. Consequently a mid-line incision was made from the base of my sternum to the top of the umbilicus. The following photograph will give you an idea of the length and location of the primary incision.

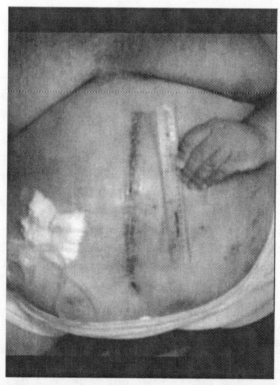

This photograph was taken 72 hours out from the commencement of the gastric bypass procedure. My weight at this time was 564 Pounds.

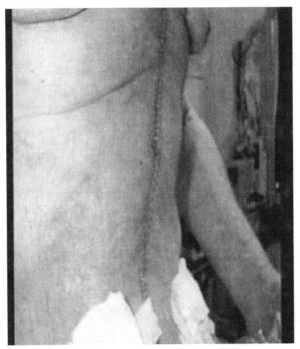

This is a photograph of what the incision looked like a week after the surgery. You'll notice that I had already started to drop a significant amount of weight! In the first week I lost about 30 pounds.

Below is a chart I developed to track my weight loss over a 15-month period.

Date	Weight	Pounds Lost	Total Pounds Lost	BMI
10/27/99	560	0	0	75.5
11/04/99	530	30	30	71.8
12/06/99	488	42	72	66.1
01/08/00	461	27	99	62.5
01/22/00	422	39	138	57.2
02/14/00	388	34	172	52.6
03/03/00	308	80	252	41.7
3/28/00	277	31	283	37.5
4/10/00	252	25	308	34.1
5/12/00	230	22	330	31.1
06/04/00	212	18	348	28.7
8/04/00	209	3	351	28.3
09/0900	190	19	370	25.7
11/109/00	177	13	383	24.0
12/10/00	162	15	398	21.9

The total, aggregate weight loss over the time period 10/99 to 12/00 was 398 Pounds !

Below are additional photographs showing what my abdomen looked like post surgery. These photos were taken over a period of about two week. So, you definitely see distinct physical changes to my body size.

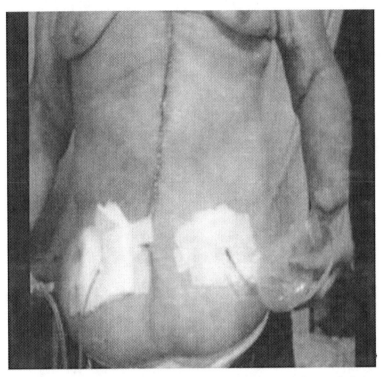

This photo was taken at week 2, prior to removal of the stainless steel staples used to close the mid line incision.
Note placement of 'drainage tubes'.

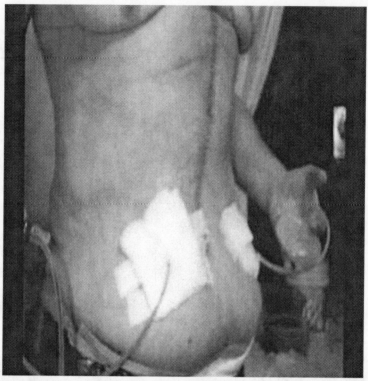

This photo is a side-view taken at week 2, prior to removal of the stainless steel staples used to close the mid line incision. Note placement of drainage tubes in panniculus

Chapter 8.
What The Doctors
Didn't Tell Me...

These are some of the specific symptoms (which risks were not revealed to me) I experienced as a result of undergoing the gastric bypass procedure. None of these things were ever mentioned to me (i.e., the possibility of these onsets). I had no idea that I might experience these symptoms and side effects of the GBS procedure:

? **Dumping syndrome**. Usually occurs when sweet foods are eaten or when food is eaten too quickly. When the food enters the small intestine, it causes cramping, sweating, and nausea. I experienced this phenomenon.

? **Abdominal hernias**. These are the most common complications requiring follow-up surgery. Incisional hernias occur in ten to twenty percent of patients and require follow-up surgery. I suffered a large Ventral Hernia post surgery which required an additional surgical procedure to close the hernia.

? **Narrowing of the stoma**. The stoma, or opening between the stomach and intestines, can sometimes become too narrow, causing vomiting. The stoma can be repaired by an outpatient procedure that uses a small endoscopic balloon to stretch it. I did not experience this phenomenon, at least to my knowledge. This can happen as a result of undergoing GBS.

? **Gallstones**. Gallstones develop in more than a third of obese patients undergoing gastric surgery. Gallstones are clumps of cholesterol and other matter that accumulate in the gallbladder. Rapid or major weight loss increases a person's risk of developing gallstones. I developed Gallstones and had to have my Gallbladder removed.

? **Leakage of stomach and intestinal contents**. Leakage of stomach and intestinal contents from the staple and suture lines into the abdomen can occur. This is a rare occurrence and sometimes seals itself. If not, another operation is required. This can result in death.

? **Acidosis**. A clinical condition wherein acid levels of bodily fluids is elevated due to over consumption of chemical based vitamin compounds. For more information see: http://www.springerlink.com/content/l625q674r02v7008/ . I experienced this phenomenon. I developed this condition resulting in the loss of twelve teeth.

? **Chemical Dependency**. According to recent studies, as many as 60% of gastric bypass patients develop chemical dependencies (addiction to analgesic drugs or alcohol) as a result of the gastric bypass surgical experience. I experienced this phenomenon with analgesics, liquid Morphine and Alcohol Addiction.

? **Personality Change**. Changes in personality are common in persons who undergo gastric bypass procedure(s). The patient is confronted with drastic changes in bodily image, changes with clothing and eating habits, and personal relationships can improve or be damaged. My personality has definitely changed. Not my attitude…but my personality. I know that I've changed…one of my undergraduate degrees is in Clinical Psychology. I've changed mentally as a function of the physical change. And my personality has changed too. It's kind of sad in a way in that I liked the guy I used to be when I was fat-obese. And people around me liked me too. I was the happy-go-lucky guy, over-indulger, live-wire and life of the party! Now, I'm very reserved and even somewhat introverted being careful to qualify and quantify every statement I might make.

????**Alcoholism and Substance Abuse** Perhaps the worst of things for which I was not prepared to deal with was the onset of Alcoholism and Substance Abuse. I reached a point during my ordeal where I seriously felt as though I was dying. I can recall sitting on the edge of my bed, vomiting blood, with my poor wife having to see all of this and listening to me cry during an extreme state of mental fugue. I was so weak and so tired of feeling the pain, and so tired of the vomiting that I honestly wanted to die. You reach a point where you just get 'tired'. Tired of the pain, tired of the vomiting, tired of not being able to do the things you used to be able to do. You miss your friends. You alienate your family members as they are now confronted with someone totally 'foreign' to them (the new person that you've become). And at times you hate yourself for what you've become (this 'new person' that *you* really don't know nor understand). And you look at your scarred body, and your new clothes and you find yourself in a state of utter cognitive dissonance! You feel 'betrayed' by the professionals; abandoned by society <and you're angry with skinny people who used to call you all of those horrible 'fat-ass' name…and kidded you…made fun of you, etc.>. At the same time you're angry at yourself for changing so radically to be like those people…who you feel caused you to go through all of the torment to loose the weight by undergoing GBS! So…you find yourself utterly confused…mad at the world and yourself for what you used to be…and for what you've become…as well as the mechanism which you feel are responsible for putting you where you are and in the condition you're in. You get angry with the practitioners whom (by) now you've decided "Don't know Shit from Apple Butter" (quote by Author). Because when you go back to them and confide to them all of these unexpected or unanticipated changes and problems you're encountering…they 'blame' you! They say you're the weak one, that the 'surgery was a success. The treatment modalities consistent were with Clinical Protocol' and that you (the patient) are responsible for your own recovery…not them! So, you decide to distance yourself from the Clinical world all together and develop the opinion that they're really 'all <just> about the dollars and the money that's made every year (telling people they're too fat and performing surgeries). You even feel more alienated (by the medical profession) because you're never asked to express your opinion(s); not asked to participate in follow-on studies and you get even more suspect when you can't get answers to your questions concerning 'Survival Rates', possible complication that might occur, and how to deal with this 'new person' into which you are about to be transformed! All of these things happened to me...and I was not prepared (mentally, physically, emotionally and socially) to deal with these things.

????**Changes in Personal and Public Relationships** WOW! This category is a ***Big One***! I can categorically and unequivocally guarantee that if you undergo GBS the nature, quality, integrity, sanctity and frequency of the quality in personal and public relationships is very definitely going to ***CHANGE*** in some manner. Every aspect of every relationship that I had prior to undergoing BPS changed after I had my surgery. Some of the changes were very positive and included improvement of the quality of life; improved physical stamina, etc. Some of these changes were negative in terms of degrees of personal disappointment. What I mean by that statement is that after I underwent the surgery and the Ordeal of Recovery I expected everyone that I knew to welcome the new Joe appreciate my new looks my improved physical condition, etc. But they didn't. At least not *everyone* in my sphere of association did. Some people I encountered a year or so after the initial surgery and recovery period said things to me like, "I liked you better when you were a Fat Slob". Or, "I don't like the way you look. You look like a Cancer Victim. You need to put some of that weight back on". Obviously those kinds of statements had their origins in *ignorance*, i.e., ignorance of what it means to *suffer from Obesity*. The people who made those statements had absolutely no idea what it was like to be "Fat" and obese in a thin-thinking society such as the Western World in the 1990's. I did not hold any grudges against those people. But I did decide that some day I would do something to educate these people in terms of coming to some understanding of obesity. And some changes have simply surprised me to the point of what I call non-expectation. I guess that in the back of my mind I must have anticipated that this kind of thing might happen thus the foresight to create a video-documentary for posterity. Perhaps the worst change came in my personal relationships with my family. Through the course of the surgery and recovery they have been subjected to witnessing sides of my personality which I never knew existed nor did I ever conceive would manifest. These included mood swings; bouts of depression; blackouts from use of prescription narcotics/pain killer; alcohol use and the list just goes on and on. Imagine for the moment that you were forced to come to terms with your physical mortality and that you finally realized that you are very sick and are probably going to be dead very soon? How does one react when faced with that realization? Does the person turn to God? Does the person turn to friends and family? How does one deal with that kind of realization given that the level of physical pain is on a scale of ten-plus? Some people could probably handle a situation like that pretty easily. Admittedly, I did not. I was scared as hell and in my mind I thought that each day was my last. For almost a year after the surgery I could not lift anything heavier than a spoon. And I could not drink more than a half ounce of any kind of fluid. The only fluids that I could tolerate and not vomit-up were liquid Morphine elixirs and one hundred proof vodkas. Before the surgery I never took a drop of alcohol: Never! The doctors and other professionals never told me anything about the possibility of developing any kind of addictions. Perhaps they just did not know at the time? I can't say for sure.

Since youth I always felt that I was immortal and that death was something that happened to people who deserved to die. That was my *logic* until I was confronted with the realization and knowledge that I had been resuscitated not once but thrice during the first surgery. And after the surgery when I started to bleed uncontrollably one day at home and my poor wife had to cleanup buckets of blood it was almost more than I could handle mentally. Although Suicide to me was and always will be out of the question there was a time when I thought that it might be better to be dead than to continue experiencing so much pain and weakness. Not to mention the Hell I putting my family through. The bullshit I put them through was horrible and so out of character for me. I did stupid things crazy things for which I am and will always be remorseful. I can recall times when I passed out as a result of intense pain. I think that the physical pain is unnecessary in today's day and age of advance Pharmacology. I could see where pain therapy back in the late Eighteen Hundreds was totally different from today's modern medical practices. Some people reading this section may form that opinion that I am some kind of wimp or have mental problems and need to grow up get a life and should have just had the intestinal fortitude to just deal with it. There will be millions of people who read these words whom are neither obese now nor will ever undergo the experience that I survived. My hope is that what I have written here will help the reader to understand how terribly debilitating obesity really is and how obesity affects every aspect of the obese person's life. These effects are far-reaching from the closest personal relationships to jobs to public facilities to the point of Societal Stigmatization which is nearly persecutory against obese people in nature in Western Society. I feel qualified to make that statement based on one of my undergraduate degrees of education. I hold a Bachelor of Arts Degree in the Social Sciences from the University of Pittsburgh. I undertook four years of comprehensive studies of peoples and cultures and studied mores, pathways and folkways of the predominant world cultures. So I can speak to this and proffer opinions based on my experience education and publication of these observations.

Unfortunately for me I experienced all but one of the above pathologies. I did not experience narrowing of the stoma. I experienced the Dumping Syndrome. I suffered a large ventral hernia of the central incision which had to be surgically repaired about a year after the initial surgery. I developed Gallstones resulting in eventual removal of the gallbladder which required another surgical procedure. Development of gallstones is common in patients who experience a rapid loss of weight. This might happen to you too if you have this type of surgery. And I suffered a gastric leak. The most alarming of these occurrences was the advent of the gastric leak. For many months post-surgery I was unable and afraid to eat anything at all. I was reluctant to eat anything as I feared development of peritonitis and infection. In addition the rapid weight loss resulted in weakness lethargy and even depression at times. I can recall looking in the mirrors and thinking about perception problems relative to my own self-image. I witnessed the shrinking of my body size from a whopping five hundred sixty pounds to a low of just one hundred sixty three pounds. I had not weighed that little since the age of about nine years. So this caused me some real mental concerns. I wondered how much more weight I would continue to lose and had a vision of myself in a coffin dead of course weighing a mere ninety eight pounds! The thought was horrifying!

During the course of onset of these conditions I developed acidosis as a result of taking too many vitamins and my saliva became very acidic. Acidosis resulted in rapid onset of tooth decay at the gum line in my oral cavity. Although I had all but two of my thirty-two original teeth when I underwent the gastric bypass procedure with onset of Acidosis the weaker and diseased teeth soon fell victims to the harsh acid in my oral cavity. Consequently I lost six teeth within the first year after the initial surgery. No one ever mentioned this prospect to me: Development of Acidosis and possible loss of my teeth as a result of taking vitamins. In my whole life with the exception of youth I never took or used any kind of manufactured vitamins. I never subscribed to Vitamin Theory and I still don't lend that school of thought much credence. But I can state with relative surety that if you take too many vitamins you run the risk of developing Acidosis like I did. So you'll want to be aware of this prospect if you undergo GBS.

I spent the first 9 months post surgery vomiting routinely. I was never told this could be a side effect of the surgery. I was unable to eat more than an ounce of anything liquid or semi-liquid. And generally I would vomit whatever I swallowed and could not hold-down any food at all.

During that time period I became quite proficient at what I called Vomiting At-Will. I was able to visually pick-out a spot on a wall or on the ground open my mouth aiming at the spot where I was focusing. And then empty the contents of my digestive track directly on that spot! During this time period I became physically very weak. And at times I was literally unable to walk or undertake any kind of physical activity: None. To help stop the vomiting I was prescribed an elixer consisting of morphine and ethyl alcohol: An elixer known as Peregoric. The elixer was highly effective in stopping the reverse-paristalsis or vomiting. The elixer also stopped the abdominal pain within seconds of being ingested. But there was a dark side to using the prescription. I became addicted to both morphine and alcohol. I had never had any problems or history of using either drugs or alcohol. But without question I became addicted to both of these over the course of what turned out to be a two-year-long recovery period. Around that same time the famous singer Willie Nelson was leading a charge to legalize the use of Marijuana for medicinal purposes. I thought about trying Marijuana to help control the pain and vomiting and as a possible way to increase appetite. I even thought about contacting Mr. Nelson in order to advise him of my support in terms of his Cause. And to take it one step further I almost bought a ranch in California and looked at some property in Montana where use of medicinal-grade marijuana is legal. I abandoned those notions simply because the morphine elixer was so easy to get. All I had to do is visit my doctor's officer vomit all over the place and during the examination and I could get as much morphine sulfate elixer that I wanted!

During the first nine months after the actual gastric bypass surgery and in view of development of secondary problems I was convinced that I was going to die. I can recall a time sitting on the edge of my bed at home where I dry-heaved so much and for so long that I filled the one-gallon garbage can which I kept bed side with blood. When that happened I called to my wife and stated that I felt like I was dying. It was pretty frightening!

So I was never told that I could or may become addicted to pain medications that needed to be prescribed. And make no mistake: I suffered a great deal of pain. Although I was informed of the apparent risks associated with the gastric bypass procedure I had no idea and no one ever mentioned anything about the possibility developing a gastric leak or gallstones or addictions to pain medications nor the probable event of hernias. The post-operative gastric leak was the most frightening event that I experienced. You can read more about possible complications associated with having the gastric bypass procedure at JAMA's URL at: http://jama.ama-assn.org/cgi/content/full/294/15/1903 . This information is pretty recent but was nonexistent at the time

I had my surgery in 1999. So this may be of value to you in making your decision whether or not to undergo this surgical procedure.

As mentioned I developed gallstones about nine months after my surgery as a result of rapid weight loss and had to have the gallbladder surgically removed. Below are a series of photographs showing some marks on my abdomen left as a result of a minimally-invasive procedure to remove the gallbladder.

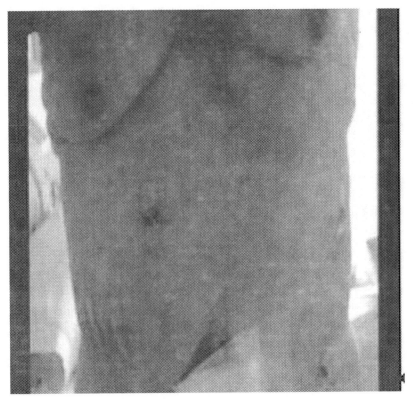

This is a photograph showing punctures as a result of minimally-invasive surgery to remove the Gallbladder.

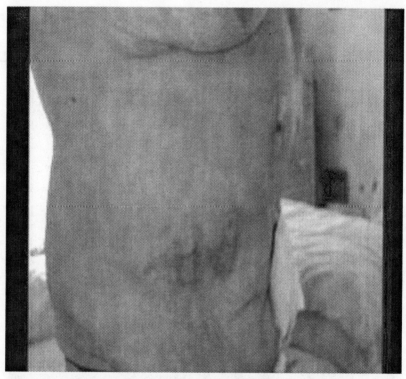

This photograph shows a right side view of my abdomen and puncture marks as a result of minimally-invasive surgery to remove the Gallbladder.

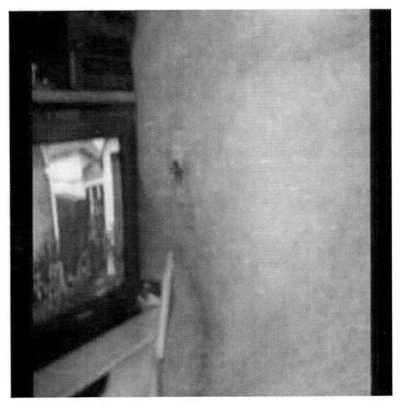

This photograph shows a left side view of my abdomen and puncture marks as a result of minimally-invasive surgery to remove the Gallbladder.

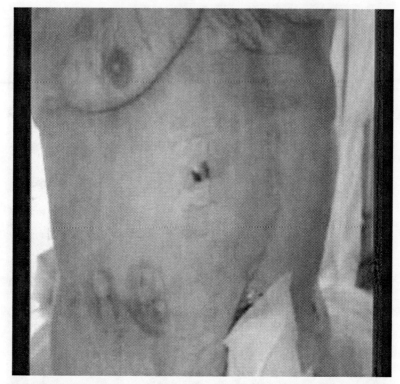

**This photograph shows a right frontal view of my abdomen and
puncture marks as a result of minimally-invasive surgery
to remove the Gallbladder.**

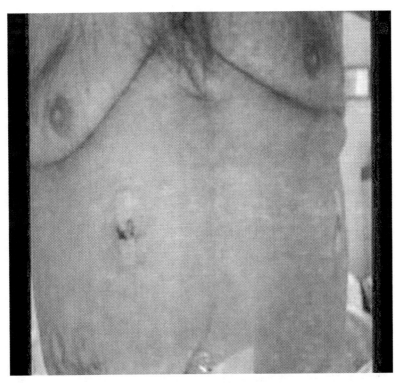

This is a full frontal view of my abdomen showing areas where the instruments were inserted into the abdomen. Note the area between the breasts comprising defect creating large, ventral hernia. The ventral hernia was eventually surgically repaired.

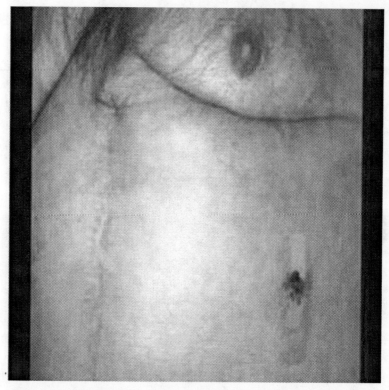

**This is a close-up view of the abdomen showing entry point
and a closer view of the ventral hernia.**

No one ever mentioned to me that my external abdominal area was going to look like a roadmap after having these surgeries. And the pain was the worst thing! I believe the worst consequence of undergoing this surgery was the incredible pain! And the vomiting as a result of the gastric leak was absolutely excruciating! For months literally I sat on the edge of my bed in my bedroom and vomited and dry-heaved into a waste basket. Due to the fact that I was advised by the nutritionist to hyper-dose on Vitamins A,B,C and D I developed Acidosis. As mentioned above this resulted in my loss of 6 teeth which literally rotted below the gum line due to the acidic nature of my saliva. I also experience mild alopecia or hair loss as a result of the Acidosis and the radical change in my blood chemistry. No one ever told me that these conditions might result. Maybe they just didn't know? Or maybe they just forgot to tell me? I can only speculate. But you should be aware of these things. In my case hyper dosing on vitamins cost me 6 teeth in the first year after my surgery. And I lost a good amount of my hair. My hair came out by the clumps. Until I finally came to the conclusion that the vitamins were doing more damage than good I stopped taking vitamins all together. I threw all of the vitamins away and to this day don't take vitamins of any kind. Although I once conversed with the late great scientist and inventor, Dr. Linus Pauling, I don't believe I gained anything from taking the vitamins and they were more of a detriment to me than beneficial. Again, to this day, I don't take vitamins nor do I concur nor subscribe to the tenets of Vitamin Theory. Be your own judge. I can only share my personal experience and observations. Based on what I've read on the subject of Vitamin Theory which is a pretty comprehensive body of knowledge as of this writing my personal belief is that use of these results only in production of vitamin-rich urine.

Perhaps the most disheartening consequence of having the surgery was my development of addiction to pain relievers and a liking for the soothing effects of liquid Morphine elixirs. I became quite adept at concocting my own formulae using one hundred proof alcohols and mixing that with the morphine sulfate I obtained under prescription from the local pharmacy. Prior to undergoing GBS I never ever drank alcohol of any kind. And I never took any kind of pain pills: None of that crap ever. And anyone who knows me can tell you that they never saw me take a drink of any kind in more than thirty years. Alcohol was just something of which I never partook. My scientific work always required me to be in absolute control of both my senses and my faculties: People's lives depended on me and my ability to make snap-decisions. So I avoided any mind-altering substances or any kind and anything that might interfere with my ability to function at or above one hundred percent! After the surgery I had my encounter with these substances. The point being that the doctors and so-called experts never warned me of the possibility of drug addiction. I've dealt with those demons and am grateful to have survived the ordeal and escaped the cycle of chasing relief from the constant agonizing pain. Today I'm pain-free. And I don't use any kind of pain relievers and I try to avoid alcohol of any kind. Developing addictions to these substances in order to relive pain is easy to do. Don't do it! Don't let yourself get trapped in this vicious cycle because it is a 'cycle' and I state from experience that addiction is a definite possible side-effect resulting from gastric bypass surgery. In fact I've thought about undertaking a study with a view toward identifying and classifying what I call the 'Post Gastric Bypass Addiction Syndrome'. This may be the first reference to such a syndrome as I have found no references to it of any of the scientific or medical literature. In the PGBAS the patient experiences all of the pathologies mentioned above with perhaps the most significant being addiction to pain medications wherein the patient becomes Alcoholic! I wanted to bring this matter to your attention because this is a very real potential outcome of the life-changes you may experience if you undergo this kind of surgery. So heads up!

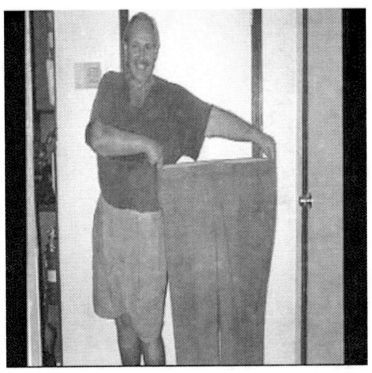

This is a photograph of me approximately 40 days after my initial gastric bypass surgery. I had already lost almost 100 Pounds!

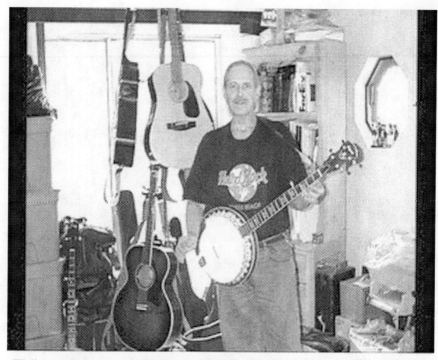

This is a photograph of what I looked liked about 3 months after my surgery. This photo was taken at my home in my Study.

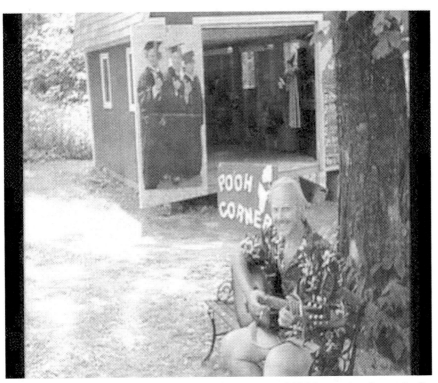

This is a photograph of me in the Summer of 2000, approximately 9 months after my gastric bypass procedure. By the Summer of 2000 I had lost nearly 350 Pounds!

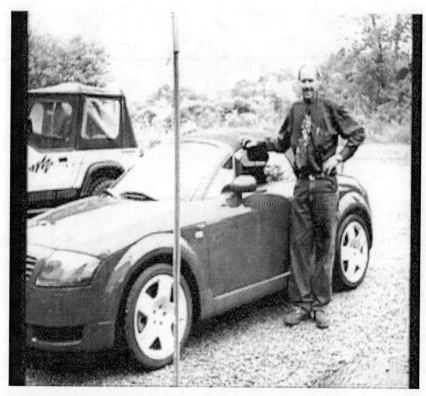

This is a photograph of me in March of 2002 at a weight of just 164 Pounds! By this time I had lost a total of 384 Pounds!

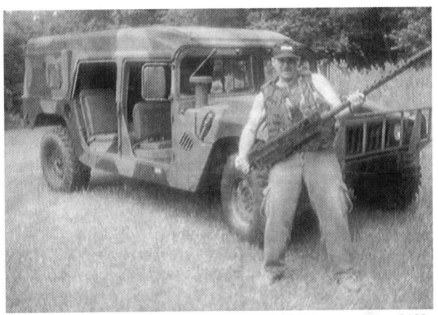

This is a photograph of me in the Summer of 2004 at a weight of 180 Pounds. I'm shown holding a 50 Caliber Machine Gun and the Humvee in the background was just fitted with a 'HotTop' I invented (see: www.necti.org)

Chapter 9.
Who Is This Guy…Anyway?

Many of you are curious to know more about me or what I may have accomplished in my life time. And you're probably wondering what makes me think I'm an expert on any subject? Certainly I can speak to the experience of undergoing the GBS losing almost four hundred pounds and then living to tell about it. So that makes me somewhat of an expert in terms of being able to speak to my own life experience with regard to this subject. But in order to assuage any preconceived concerns and to satisfy what I consider to be a natural curiosity I've decided to include a copy of the biographical sketch and the resume that both NASA and the Federal Bureau of Investigation have in their files regarding my background. My hope is that you gain some additional insights about me via this information.

Biographical Sketch
Dr. Joseph A. Resnick, PhD

Dr. Joseph A. Resnick began his professional career in 1972 at the age of 19 years at which time he accepted an employment position in the Maintenance Department at Westinghouse Electric & Manufacturing Corporation's East Pittsburgh Pennsylvania World Headquarters, as a 'Sweeper'. Several months later Dr. Resnick was recruited into The Westinghouse Technical School Corporate Apprentice Program.

Between the time periods 1974 thru 1976, he attained Associate Science Degrees in both Electrical and Mechanical Engineer and a certification in a new field, called, "Electro-Mechanical Robotics'. During that time, Dr. Resnick received various security clearances enabling him to work on special projects for the US Navy, US Dept. of Energy, The Nuclear Regulatory Commission and the US Army. In 1978 Dr. Resnick was assigned to duties at Westinghouse in the Long-Range Major Development Laboratory (MD-X-Lab) where he participated in experiments with 1.5 Kv VanDeGraff Generators, SF-6Kv Gas-Fired Circuit Breaker Systems and a special project involving Electro-Motive Force Weapons now commonly referred to as 'Rail Guns'. Dr. Resnick is considered to be a world authority regarding Electro-Motive-Force or EMF-weapons systems.

In 1979 Dr. Resnick separated from Westinghouse Electric Corporation and returned to college as a full time student at the University of Pittsburgh in Pittsburgh, Pennsylvania where he studied Medicine and BioMechanical Engineering. Studies at the University of Pittsburgh led to his initial filing of numerous US and Foreign Patent Applications related to implantable hearing and speech devices while working on projects such as the Jarvik-V and VII (artificial heart designs), the artificial kidney (pump), and his own artificial human speech devices being developed at the University of Pittsburgh's School of Medicine. His earliest success came in 1983 with his development of a design entitled, In-The-Ear Talk-Though Hearing Protection Device, for the US Army. The patent and development rights were licensed with that early design evolving into what is known and marketed today as micro-sized hearing aids. Subsequently, Resnick designed and patented a number of various artificial human speech restoration devices. One device comprised a palatal element technology which evolved into a sophisticated telemetry and armament command system used in aircraft fighters which may still be in use. That technology was used during the Falkland Islands War...resulting in the loss of the entire Chilean Air Force in less than thirteen minutes! You may examine Dr. Resnick's US Patent #

6,272,781 related to 'Wearable Counter-Measure Devices' and Reactive Body Armor systems where voiced and non-voiced control systems are still in use today. The US Army calls these kinds of technologies, 'Future Soldier Systems'.

It was during this time period (1982-1986) that Dr. Resnick developed an affiliation with NASA and was assigned to various projects resulting in design of systems and sub-systems for the STS Shuttle Fleet, including on-board fueling and fluid recovery systems, as well as the waste elimination systems and sub-system for use in space suits (by ILC Dover). Dr. Resnick, in collaboration with a Canadian Colleague developed the first 'Exo-Skeletal Exercise Suit' which was designed to circumvent the onset of Fluid Drift in humans in microgravity conditions during orbit. The device was submitted to NASA Johnson Space Flight Center for consideration. NASA opted to use a treadmill device designed by NASA scientist, Dr. William Thornton, with whom Dr. Resnick collaborated. The Exo-Skeletal Exercise suits designed by Dr. Resnick were later adapted by the US Air Force for use in what we know today as Anti-G-Suits which prevent loss of consciousness by pilots during +6-G maneuvers. Dr. Resnick is one of the Founding Members of the Aerospace Medical Association's Human Factors Engineering Branch.

Dr. Resnick was invited by NASA to exhibit seven of his discoveries at NASA's Kennedy Space Center, Florida in the Galaxy Arcade where these appeared from the time period 1985 thru 1995. In cooperation with a request from NASA's Technology Transfer Program, Dr. Resnick capitulated and a display was created and located next to the Moon Rocks Exhibit at Kennedy Space Center. The display included the Resnick Tone Emitter (artificial/computerized human speech devices); The PAS-45 (Pollution Alert System with .45 micron filters used in space suits); The Resnick Speech Teachers (wrist-mounted and clinician's models); Artificial Human Sweat Glands comprising .25um glass microspheres; and the first medical instrument designed to be used in Space by Astronauts and crews, the 'ECADD'

(Electronic Cleansing and Debridement Device). If you visited the Kennedy Space Center in Florida during that time period and saw the Moon Rock Exhibit you saw Dr. Resnick's discoveries.

From the years 1986-1991 Dr. Resnick worked special initiatives for various Department of Defense initiatives related to development of low-observable technologies resulting in the issuance of **US Patent 5,163, 504, Container Heating or Cooling Device and Novel Building Material, and US Patent Number 5,523,757, Signal Dampening Camouflage System.** Technologies reduced to practice in these patents played a critical part in the early victories enjoyed by Allied Forces and the USA prior to and during Operation Desert Storm. You may recognize tenets of the Signal Dampening System today in movies such as "Predator" which shows an Alien creature with the ability to blend into backgrounds and become 'invisible'. Or, you may find this technology in the oceans on ships or in the air on special kinds of aircraft or on phased-array antenna systems in programs such as HAARP.

During the time period 1989-1996, Dr. Resnick's research activities focused on further refinement of microencapsulation instrumentation, live cell encapsulation methodologies. At about the same time Dr. R. Buckminster Fuller conceptualized 'Buckey-Balls', Dr. Resnick configured an apparatus using a second-hand pressure cooker which he and his wife purchased at a church rummage sale. With some modifications using Visqueen tubing and syringes of various sizes the first 'nanocapsules' were produced at Dr. Resnick's laboratory in rural Fawn Township Pennsylvania. This capability was first disclosed in the US Patent Application which resulted in the issuance of US Patent # 5,163,504 which had originally contained 123 Claims in the Parent Application but was held in abeyance by the 902 Section at the United States Patent Office for six years. The application was eventually permitted to issue with a limited number of published Claims.

At the time of the Crash of the Exxon Valdez on March 24, 1989, Dr. Resnick was completing studies for attainment of a Master's Degree as NASA Scholar at the Military College of Vermont. Dr. Resnick lived for a short time with his wife and family in Sarasota, Florida. At that time, Dr. Resnick was employed as an Environmental Specialist III for Sarasota County Government BCC where he was completing an Externship in a position that had been arranged through recommendation of Dr. Resnick's Academic Adviser, a high-place Official at NASA. In actuality, Dr. Resnick was engaged in research on a special initiative involving compromise of the 'Stealth Coatings' used in the F-117 air platforms Stealth Fighters which had been detected by Israeli Radar Systems some 6 months prior to the commencement of Operation Desert Storm. Based on NASA's familiarity with Dr. Resnick's expertise in fabrication of microstructures and microclimates Resnick was asked to solve the problem for the DoD. Dr. Resnick was able to solve the problem of peeling flaking of the RAM (Radar-Attenuating Materials) and a test was conducted with the newly developed materials at the Chicago White Sox Farm League Stadium in late 1989. A copy of the videotape showing tests utilizing a hand-held radar gun (16.25 GHz range) in the Locker Room of the Chicago White Sox Stadium is on deposit in the Library at Vermont College in Montpelier, VT, and likewise Registered with the US Copyright Office in Washington, DC (available on records and in Braille). While living in Florida and in his spare time Dr. Resnick developed three new species of Sea Grasses utilizing gene-splicing techniques he developed. This research was undertaken in an effort to counter the demise of indigenous sea grasses which serve as the main food sources for the West Indian Manatee (*Tricacus manatus*).

With the crash of the Exxon Valdez in 1989 Dr. Resnick set about to utilize his ability to make microspheres with a view toward utilizing this capability to assist in the clean-up of Prince William Sound. Dr. Resnick's efforts led to development of a family of novel bioremediation tools (see www petrolrem.com), such as PRP

(Petroleum Remediation Product), Bio-Boom, Bio-Sok, Oil-Buster, Poly-Sorbe and Micro-Sorbe (all product names Trademark Claimed by Dr. Resnick), which are in worldwide use, today and marketed through a company he helped to found. In September 1994, NASA spotlighted Dr. Resnick's accomplishments by featuring him on the cover of its national publication, NASA TECH BRIEFS, in a story entitled, "MISSION ACCOMPLISHED". The story in NASA Tech Briefs details Dr. Resnick's development of bioremediation technologies. In 1996, Dr. Resnick's technology was placed in the SPINOFF NASA HALL OF FAME.

From the time period 1991-2001, Dr. Resnick participated in numerous projects for various DoD components both in the USA and abroad.

In October 2001, several weeks after the events of September 11, 2001, Dr. Resnick left his employment position as Chief Scientist with PetrolRem, Inc. to undertake efforts to develop next-generation future soldier systems based on US Patent # 6,272,781. Since that time Dr. Resnick has served as Chief Scientist for NxGenUSA Corporation, NxGenBodyArmorUSA and Up-ArmorUSA Corporation of Pittsburgh, PA and Alexandria, VA. In this capacity Dr. Resnick heads up all R&D efforts in the Future Soldier Systems Divisions and the Vehicle Up-Armor Divisions at various locations throughout the USA, Canada, South America, and Europe. In addition to these duties, Dr. Resnick functions as Chief Scientist for various projects for the U.S. Department of the Interior, The US Department of Energy, The Bureau of Land Management, NASA, the US ARMY ARL, SAALT, APG and TACOM. In several of the above projects, Dr. Resnick collaborates with a team comprising world-renowned experts in the area of ion propagation sciences for programs such as HAARP. Dr. Resnick and his team are consultants to His Majesty, King Abdullah II of Jordan in various initiatives related to low-observable technologies and Multi-National Security initiatives.

In September 2004, at the request of several Scientific Directorates in the Nation's Capitol, Dr. Resnick was asked to undertake the stand-up of a new Domestic Counter-Terrorism Center. In October 2004, Dr. Resnick, with support of private citizens, enabled the stand-up of the National Anti-Terrorism Technology Development and Training Center ('NAT2DTC"). NAT2DTC has recently formed the National Eco-Counter Terrorism Center and Institute (see: WWW.NECTI.Org).

The following is a list of Dr. Resnick's accomplishments to date:

PUBLICATIONS

PATENT ISSUED TITLE

US0627278108/14/2001 Close-Contact Counter-Measure Garment/Method

US0580772409/15/1998 Degradation of petroleum hydrocarbons with organisms encapsulated in wax

US0552375706/041996 Signal dampening camouflage system and manufacturing method (Stealth/Aircraft Coatings)

US0516350411/17/1992 Container heating or cooling device and building material

US0505214610/01/1991 Fishing equipment

US0501517905/14/1991 Speech monitor

US0470629211/10/1987 Speech prosthesis

US0457173902/18/1986 Interoral Electrolarynx

US0442491101/10/1984 Container Tamper-Detection Device/Method

Can022124 07/09/1987 Interoral Speech Prosthesis (Computerized-interface)

Swe037718 08/04/1987 Interoral Speech Prosthesis (Computerized-interface)

WPO07911 02/18/1986 Interoral Electrolarynx (Palatal Element with Power Supply)

Classified (In-the-ear Talk-through Hearing Protection Device)
Classified (Intra-Oral Telemetry Control Device)
Classified (Voice/Non-voiced Systems Command Device)
Classified (Palatal-element switch)
Classified (Ocular Sighting Means/Method)

NASA Tech Briefs, Cover Story, September, 1994 ("Mission Accomplished"). Contact Ms. Linda Bell, Editor-In-Chief, NASA Tech Briefs Magazine, NY, NY, Email to: Linda.Bell@abptuf.org for information.

Exhibitor of 7 Inventions in Galaxy Arcade, NASA Kennedy Space Center, Florida, 1986-1996.

PATENTS PENDING APPROVAL

SERIAL NUMBERFILING DATE TITLE

S.N.08021199 00000 1998 Entomological Treatment and Method (Bee Medica for treatment of varrowa and
tracheal mites in feral Bee and Honey Bee populations)

S.N.099889 00000 1998 Photographic Counter-measure Device and Method (*Paparazzi Stopper?*)

S.N.4402-1 00000 1999 Controlled-Burn, Self-Extinguishing Igniter

S.N.655545 00000 1998 Anti-Bacterial Packaging with Contamination Indicator (color-change)

S.N. 83322 00000 1999 Remote-Sensing Counter-Measure Garment and Method of Counter-Counter Measure from Chem-Bio-Nuclear Attack

(USPO 902 Section Pending Classification)

S.N.129909 0000 1997 Self-Sterilizing Counter-top

S.N. 55545 0000 1997 Hand-Held Portable Food Sterilizer

S.N. 42233 0000 2001 Delivery System/Method for Counter-Measure of Biological WMD's (Weapons of Mass Destruction)

S.N. 42234 0000 2001 Method/Apparatus for Biological Decontamination of Containers, Foodstuffs, Clothing and US Mails (Unsolicited Proposal Pending to US Postal Service)

S.N. 42235 0000 2001Interactive Defense System/Method for Aircraft, Conveyances and the Home

S.N. 42236 0000 2001 Manufacturing Method/Apparatus for Biological, Chemical and Nuclear Weapons of Mass Destruction "WMD's" (902 Section Pending Classification)

S.N. 42237 0000 2003 Inter-Oral Telemetry Control and Switching Means/Method/Apparatus for High-Speed Aircraft and Weaponry Systems

S.N. 42238 0000 2003 Physiological/Galvanometric Power Supply, Switching Means, Method and Apparatus

S.N. 03773 0602 2002 Transverse Reflective-Protective Contact Eye Lenses and Coatings for Conventional Face-Mounted Apparatus, Manufacturing Method and Kit

S.N. 47882 0212 2000 Mammalian Collision-Avoidance Device for *Tricacus manatus* (West Indian Manatee)

S.N. 69966 0519 2000 Novel Genetic-sequence and Species of (3) Indigenous Sea grasses Common to Gulf of Mexico, Caribbean Sea and Atlantic Ocean (Gene-Spl Recomb DNA Method)

See "WWW.USPTO.gov" for a complete listing of issued U.S. and Foreign Patents.

See "WWW.USPTO.gov/Copyrights" for a complete list of Copyrighted publications.

Other Patents Pending or Filed as Applications:

1. Electronic ID Tag using RFID for Humans, K-9's Horses

2. Public Identity Portal (Public Telephones with Biometric, Voice Print/Iris-Scan Identification systems and method of use in public places)

3. RFID-Read-Write Chip used in Cell-Phones

4. NexTrem Body Armor (for extremities)

5. Rapid-Deployable Vehicle Up Armor Kits

6. Next-Generation Up-Armor Encapsulation Method and Means for Short Cargo Bed Covers for HMMWV's and LAV's

7. Fractal Geometric Pattern Designs for Visual Mitigation of Architectures, Structures and Conveyances

8. Food Storage Containers with Dental Appliance Contained

9. Passive I-R Counter-Measure Garment and Method

Last Update: 5/10/06

Conclusion

My sincere hope is that what I have presented above helps you, the Reader, in some way. This *Help* might take the form of building your confidence or better preparing you to face what is certain to be the most challenging ordeal in your lifetime if you choose to undergo this kind of surgery. I consider myself to be extremely fortunate to have both survived the ordeal, lived to tell about it, keep the weight off, and enjoy life to the fullest every day! Please take some time to acquire the video presentation, *"You Can Live Again"* (US Copyright # PA-1-012-307, Nov 02, 2000) which may be obtained by contacting me through my website at www.publishamerica.com . I invite you to visit the following URL where you can find additional information about an exercise device I invented and developed for morbidly obese people. I used this device to aid me in my recovery. Please see: http://www.geocities.com/jreznik888/photopagespiral.html. Finally, if I were able to give something to everyone who might read this book and who watches the video presentation that gift would be gift of Hope for a better quality of life.

—*Dr. Joseph A. Resnick, Inventor*

Printed in the United States
117613LV00005B/351/A